Vegan Recipes

The Ultimate Step-by-Step Illustrated Guide for Beginners to Cook Easy, Tasty and Healthy Meals Based on the Vegan Diet. Plant-Based Recipes On a Budget

HOWIE DYSON

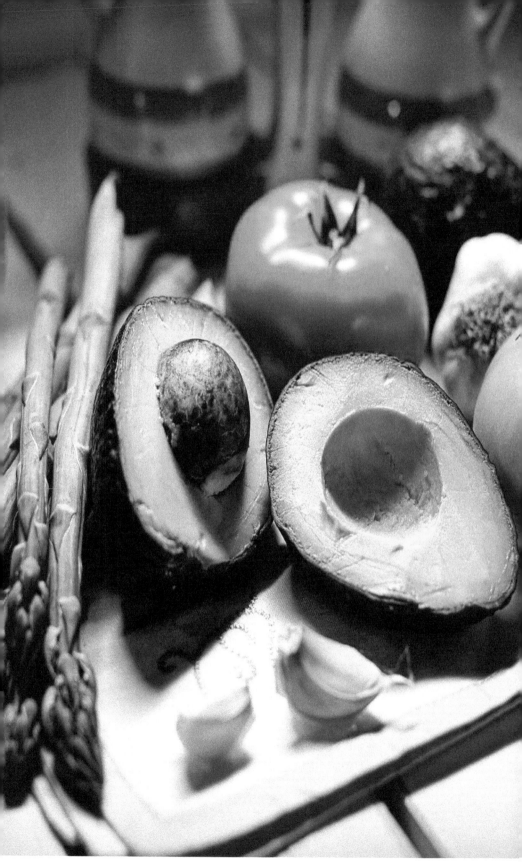

Table of Content

Introduction

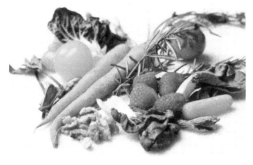

The vegan diet, not to be confused with a vegetarian diet, has become more and more popular over the years. Unlike other diets, the vegan diet has little to do with calories and carbs. A vegan diet completely restricts the consumption of animal products. Many individuals come to the vegan diet for various reasons that usually fall into three categories: health, ethical, and environmental. Eating a vegan, plant-based diet can dramatically improve issues or problems in all three categories. This section will discuss the health problems associated with eating meat and dairy, the damage it's doing to the environment, and ethical issues surrounding the meat and dairy industry. In addition, we'll tell you everything you need to know about fish and eggs. Fish and eggs are not a part of a vegan diet, and after seeing the research, eliminating them will be easy. This section will be crucial in understanding why the consumption of animal products is not suitable for everyday life and why it's best to eliminate them.

Why Vegan

Deciding to live a vegan lifestyle likely was influenced by information regarding personal health, ethical reasons, or growing environmental problems. Veganism has a hand in each of these categories and can significantly improve the quality of life in individuals, animals, and the planet. As the population grows, so does the demand to produce food. Farmers and industries feel the pressure to produce mass quantities of product as quickly as possible. Unfortunately, many products are produced at the cost of your health, the well-being of animals, and the environment. Many studies have emerged in regard to plant-based diets versus meat/cheese diets. As technology progresses, more and more information becomes accessible to the public. Although many of these studies aren't promoted, they're out there and large companies do their best to confuse the American public. The reasons to switch to a plant-based diet are ever growing, but this section will highlight what you need to know.

Health

In regard to health, a vegan diet contains the best foods for the human body. A vegan diet is nutrient rich and relies on whole grains, fruits, vegetables, beans, legumes, nuts, and seeds for nutrition. These foods, bought organically, only contain minerals and vitamins that promote the health of the body. According to a study by the Federal Commission for Nutrition (Battaglia Richi et al., 2015), meat is associated with an increased risk of total mortality, which takes into consideration the likelihood of developing diseases like cardiovascular disease, colorectal cancer, and type 2 diabetes. With so many companies and advertisements promoting the consumption of meat, you may be scratching your head. The truth is numerous science-based studies have come out over the past decade showing the effect meat has on the body.

Processed meats like sausages, hot dogs, salami, ham, bacon, beef jerky, and canned meat are considered type one carcinogens according to The World Health Organization (2015). A type one carcinogen means that there is sufficient evidence that the agent causes cancer. These meats fall into the same category as tobacco and asbestos, which are known for their toxicity to the human body.

There is a known connection between meat and diabetes. One serving of processed meat daily increases the risk of developing diabetes by 51% according to a study (Micha, Michas, & Mozaffarian, 2012). Diabetes is a disease that many are familiar with. According to the National Diabetes Federation (2019), it's estimated that 515 million people suffer from diabetes worldwide, which equates to 1 in 11 adults. Not only is this unfortunate for those suffering from the disease but also for taxpayers as one of three Medicare dollars is spent on people with diabetes (Cubanksi, Neuman, True, & Damico, 2019). The money spent on diabetes yearly is staggering. Cardiovascular diseases are also on the rise. Over 17 million people die every year from cardiovascular disease, making it the number one cause of death globally (World Health Organization, 2017). To put this into perspective, the amount of people who die from cardiovascular disease is the equivalent of four jumbo jets crashing every single hour, every day, every single year according to the popular documentary *What the Health* (n.d.). With so many deaths from cardiovascular disease, extensive funding has gone into studies to try and expose the reason behind the drastic growth. The health of arteries, cholesterol, unhealthy fats, and sodium all play a role in heart complications. With the number one dietary source of cholesterol being chicken, new studies have challenged the nutrition of chicken (Drewnowski & Rehm, 2013). Although many thought chicken was a safer alternative to eating red meat, it turns out chicken contains the same components that will cause high levels of blood cholesterol (National Heart, Lung, and Blood Institute, 2019).With all the health complications, cancer is always a hot topic. It's likely you or someone you know has suffered from a type of cancer or multiple types. Cancer is a word no one ever likes to hear or discuss, for good reason. Most of the general public would do anything to avoid cancer in any form. When most of us think about being healthy, fitness and prevention of disease comes to mind. What many don't know is that daily habits are taking a toll on our fitness without us even knowing. As information gets out and people spread the world, it can be hard to decipher facts from propaganda. This is where scientific studies come in handy. Dairy is linked to prostate cancer, breast cancer, colon cancer, autoimmune diseases, and more. Dairy products contain hormones that the body registers as unnatural. Milk proteins from cows are completely different and contain high levels of animal protein. According to a study, for women who have had breast cancer, just one serving of dairy a day can increase their chances from dying from breast cancer by 49%, and dying from any disease 64% (Kroenke et al., 2013). For men, eating dairy can increase the likelihood of getting prostate cancer by 34% (Physicians Committee for Responsible Medicine, n.d.). These statistics are alarming, and these studies are out there even though you won't see them advertised by McDonald's, Burger King, or Pizza Hut. Because it's hard to truly know what's being put into food, it's likely most of the meat being consumed has some type of unnatural substances. Animals are often treated for any diseases they acquire, and we truly don't know what they are eating/drinking. Animals living in congested areas are exposed to diseases, fecal matter, bacteria, and germs, many of which stay in their blood steam. In a Retail Meat Report, performed by the Federal Drug and Administration (2010), test results showed 88% of pork chops, 90% of ground beef, and 95% of chicken breasts that were sampled were contaminated with fecal bacteria. and a study by Hernández et al. (2015) confirmed that even buying organic meat does not diminish the carcinogenic potential in terms of persistent organic pollutants (POPs). The study took organic and conventional meats of all sorts and tested them on a group of voluntary, Spanish participants. The study showed little differences between organic and conventional meats in regard to their carcinogenic/contaminated nature. The difference between the two meats was minimal, and Hernández, goes on to say that organic labels are overused as propaganda in the meat industry. In reality, the exposure to toxins is pretty much the same in regard to organic vs. not organic. Another common issue the American public is struggling with is weight. Excess weight causes complications within the body and prevents the body from functioning properly. In the United States, two thirds of adults are overweight or obese (National Institute of Diabetes and Digestive and Kidney Diseases, 2017). Complex carbs and natural sugars have been looped into the idea that they're unhealthy and cause weight gain. In reality, empty calories, and low fat and low nutrient foods have taken oven the American eye. With the surplus of advertising from hundreds of food/restaurant chains, good healthy eating has been put on the back burner. However, a vegan diet has shown impressive numbers in regard to weight. One study by the Physicians Committee for Responsible Medicine (2018) found vegan subjects to have lower cholesterol levels, triglycerides, blood pressure, and a lower overall Body Mass Index (BMI) in comparison to the meat eating subjects. Switching to a vegan diet doesn't have to be difficult as many of the same foods can still be enjoyed with healthy moderations.

Environment

With mass production of meat, the environment is taking a beating. Raising and fattening up animals for better profit comes at a cost. Raising animals for food is the leading cause of rainforest destruction, species extinction, ocean dead zones, and fresh water consumption according to the documentary *What the Health* (A. U. M. Films, 2019). Another topic frequently discussed is the effect of carbon dioxide and its impact on the environment. You may be surprised to know that raising animals for consumption produces more greenhouse gases than the entire transportation sector (Food and Agriculture Organization of the United Nations, n.d.). This statistic takes into consideration the pollution given off by cars, trains, ships, airplanes, buses, and cargo ships. Greenhouse gases are dangerous because they disrupt normal ecosystem functions. Global warming is a hot topic and coincides with the effects greenhouse gases have on the environment. Below are a few of the disturbing statistics that illuminate the problems of the current meat and dairy industry:

- A car would have to drive 200 miles (320 km) to emit the same amount of emissions as one single burger containing 0.5lbs (200 g) of meat (Food Engineering, 2012).

- Huge areas of rainforest are cleared for the supply of animal feed and for pastureland; the CO_2 emission soars to 335 kg for one kilogram of beef (Food Engineering, 2012).

- Studies show that going vegan can cut an individual's personal carbon footprint in half (Mercy for Animals, 2014).

- McGill University and the University of Minnesota (2012) explained the relationship with meat production and world hunger. Humans actually produce enough grain to feed the world, but we choose to feed most of it to animals just so we can eat meat (Seufert, Ramankutty, & Foley, 2012).

- Animal agriculture is responsible for two thirds of all freshwater consumption in the world today (Florio, 2015).

Ethical

Many vegans will say this is the number one reason they were first attracted to the lifestyle. Many of the animals killed and produced for meat are intelligent and have similar feelings to humans. Pigs, cows, chickens, and hens are all treated poorly by the meat industry. The meat industry is a business and in order to make a high profit, animal comfort is the first thing thrown out the door. Hundreds of thousands of animals are packed into tiny living quarters where they develop diseases and illnesses and are exposed to massive amounts of fecal material. When thinking about this, you may realize that it would be impossible to keep a clean facility with the number of animals living there. Per Food Safety News (Loglisci, 2010), "According to new data just released by the Food and Drug Administration (FDA), of the antibiotics sold in 2009 for both people and food animals almost 80% were reserved for livestock and poultry." Considering the pharmaceutical industry sells 80% of antibiotics made to animal agriculture, you could say that keeping animals healthy in these facilities is near impossible. These intelligent animals don't have a good quality of life.

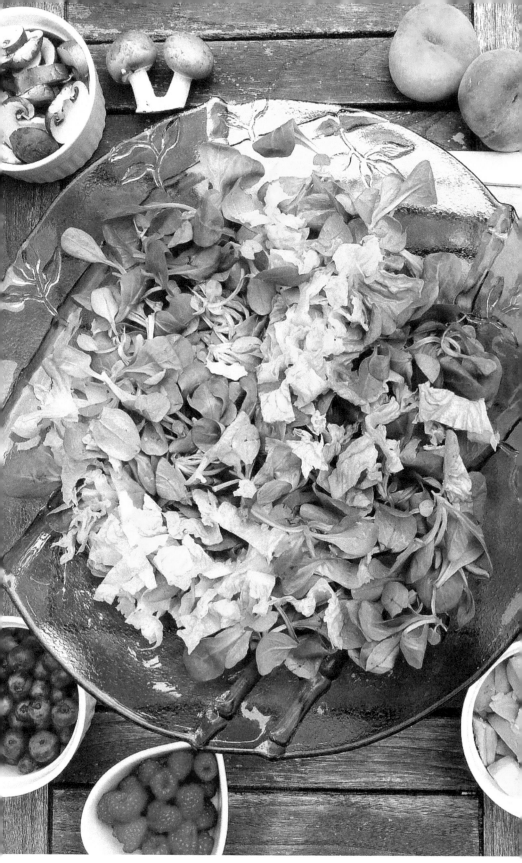

Breakfast Recipes

Below are the recipes for breakfast, lunch, and dinner.

Breakfast One - Breakfast Hash

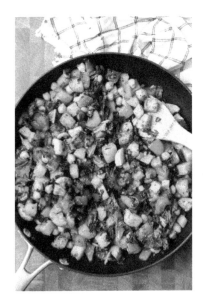

Nutritional Information Per Serving:

280 Calories, 10 grams of Fat, 36 grams of Carbs, 6 grams of Protein

Time: 20 minutes

Serving Size: 3 servings

Ingredients:

- 3 medium potatoes, diced
- 1 cup onion, chopped
- 1 medium red bell pepper, chopped
- 1 cups mushrooms, sliced
- 1 teaspoon spices of choice (garlic, cumin, paprika, or combo)
- 2 tablespoons avocado oil
- Himalayan salt and pepper to preference

Directions:

1. In a medium skillet, pour and mix avocado oil and potatoes.

2. Sauté on medium heat until potatoes are soft or slightly crispy.

3. Add in other vegetables and spices.

4. Sauté until vegetables are soft.

Breakfast Two - Breakfast Cookies

Nutritional Information Per Cookie: 207 Calories, 12 grams of fat, 24 grams of carbs, 5 grams of protein

Time: 15 minutes

Serving Size: 8 cookies

Ingredients:

- 1 cup old fashioned rolled oats

- ½ cup oat flour

- ½ cup dried cranberries

- ½ cup pepitas, unsalted

- ¼ cup ground flax seed

- 1 tablespoon of chia seeds

- 1 teaspoon cinnamon

- ½ teaspoon baking powder

- generous pinch of Himalayan salt

- 1 large banana, mashed

- 3 tablespoons melted coconut oil

- 2 tablespoons almond milk, unsweetened

Directions:

1. Preheat oven to 375 Fahrenheit or 190 degrees Celsius. Line a baking sheet with parchment paper.

2. Combine all dry ingredients in a large mixing bowl and mix well.

3. Stir in banana, coconut oil, and almond milk.

4. Let the mixture sit for 5 minutes.

5. Start scooping the mixture and form a small ball. Place ball on lined baking sheet and press to flatten into cookies.

6. Bake for 16 minutes or until the edges of the cookies are golden.

Breakfast Three - Protein Shake: Vanilla Cashew

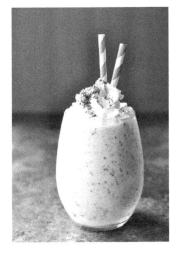

Nutritional Information Per Serving: 450 Calories, 26 grams of Fat, 45 grams of Carbs, 15 grams of Protein

Time: 5 minutes

Serving Size: 1 serving

Ingredients:

- 1 banana

- ¼ cup raw cashews

- 1 cup almond milk, unsweetened

- 1 tablespoon cashew butter (or peanut butter)

- 1 tablespoon of chia seeds

- ½ teaspoon vanilla extract

- ½ cup ice cubes

Directions:

1. Place all ingredients in a high-powered blender and blend until smooth.

Breakfast Four - Zucchini Pancakes

Nutritional Information Per Serving: 192 Calories, 7 grams of Fat, 24 grams of Carbs, 7 grams of Protein

Time: 12 minutes

Serving Size: 2 servings

Ingredients:

- ½ cup chickpea flour, sifted/lump free

- ½ cup water

- 3 teaspoons avocado oil

- 2 cups zucchini, coarsely grated

- Himalayan salt and black pepper to preference

Directions:

1. In a medium bowl, mix flour, water, salt, salt, pepper, and 1 teaspoon of avocado oil. Mix until smooth or until the batter has no lumps.

2. Add in zucchini. Stir.

3. Add 1 teaspoon of oil in a nonstick skillet and warm over medium heat. Pour in half of the batter and cook for five minutes.

4. Carefully flip the pancake and cook for an additional four minutes or until the center appears golden brown.

5. Follow steps three and four to cook the remaining pancake.

Breakfast Five - High Protein Pudding

Nutritional Information Per Serving: 455 Calories, 24 grams of Fat, 53 grams of Carbs, 55 grams of Protein

Time: 5 minutes prep, (overnight recipe)

Serving Size: 2 servings

Ingredients:

- ½ cup buckwheat groats, dry

- 2 scoops vegan pea protein powder

- 1 banana

- ½ cup oat milk

- 2 tablespoons natural almond butter (substitute a different nut butter if preferred)

- 2 teaspoons cinnamon (optional)

Directions:

1. Add the groats to a bowl and cover with water. Soak the oats overnight.

2. Use a strainer to remove water.

3. Place all ingredients, including the groats, in a high-speed blender and blend until smooth.

4. Serve immediately and add additional toppings if desired.

Breakfast Six - Breakfast Tacos

Nutritional Information Per Taco: 166 Calories, 23 grams of Fat, 20 grams of Carbs, 10 grams of Protein

Time: 10 minutes

Serving Size: 4 tacos

Ingredients:

Taco Ingredients:

- ½ cup black beans, (no salt added/low sodium)

- ½ cup salsa

- ½ medium avocado

- 4 corn tortillas

For the Eggs:

- 6 ounces block tofu, firm and drained

- ½ tablespoon olive oil

- ½ teaspoon turmeric

- 1 tablespoon nutritional yeast

- 1 tablespoon water

- sea salt and black pepper to preference

Directions:

1. To prepare the tofu eggs, pour olive oil into a skillet and warm over medium heat for one minute.

2. Add the tofu the skillet and mash into crumbles using a spatula.

3. Stir and cook tofu for 5 minutes or until most of the water is gone.

4. Add the remaining tofu ingredients and stir.

5. Prepare the tacos using the taco ingredients and tofu eggs.

Breakfast Seven - Blueberry Muffins

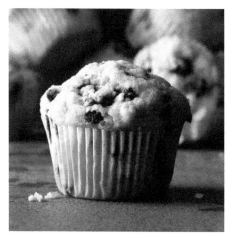

Nutritional Information Per Muffin: 218 Calories, 7 grams of Fat, 34 grams of Carbs, 4 grams of Protein

Time: 35 minutes

Serving Size: 12 muffins

Ingredients:

- 1 ¼ cup almond milk, unsweetened

- 1 teaspoon apple cider vinegar

- 2 cups whole wheat pastry flour

- 2 tablespoons Stevia powder (2 teaspoons Stevia drops)

- 2 teaspoons baking powder

- 1 tablespoon cornstarch

- ⅓ cup melted coconut oil

- 1 teaspoon vanilla extract

- 1½ cups blueberries

Directions:

1. Preheat oven to 400 Fahrenheit or 205 Celsius. Line muffin pan with liners and lightly spray them with oil.

2. Combine almond milk and apple cider vinegar in a cup and set aside.

3. In a large mixing bowl, combine and mix all dry ingredients. Pour in the almond milk and apple cider vinegar mixture.

4. Add coconut oil and vinegar to the large mixing bowl.

5. Fold in blueberries.

6. Divide mixture evenly into the 12 liners.

7. Bake for 20-25 minutes or until the top is golden brown. Use a toothpick and wait to remove muffins until it comes out clean after being placed in the center.

8. Allow cooling and use an airtight container to store in the refrigerator or freezer.

Breakfast Eight - Green Smoothie

Nutritional Information Per Serving: 410 Calories, 21 grams of Fat, 58 grams of Carbs, 4 grams of Protein

Time: 5 minutes

Serving Size: 1 serving

Ingredients:

- 1 medium sized banana

- 2 cups of fresh spinach

- ½ avocado

- 2 cups coconut milk, unsweetened

- 1 medium sized apple (remove core)

- 1 cup of ice

- cold water as needed/to preference

Directions:

1. Add all ingredients to a high-powered blender and blend until smooth.

Breakfast Nine - Bread Recipe, One

Nutritional Information Per Serving: 191 Calories, 12 grams of Fat, 16 grams of Carbs, 6 grams of Protein

Time: 1 hour 15 minutes

Serving Size: 15 servings

Ingredients:

- 2 cups rolled oats

- 5 tablespoons psyllium husks

- 1 cup sunflower seeds

- 2 tablespoons pepitas

- 2 tablespoons almonds, whole

- 2 tablespoons hazelnuts, whole

- ½ cup and 1 tablespoon ground flax seeds

- 2½ tablespoons chia seeds

- ½ teaspoon Himalayan salt

- 1½ teaspoon coconut oil

- 1¾ cups warm water

Directions:

1. In a large bowl, combine all ingredients. Mix well.

2. Cover the mixing bowl and refrigerate overnight.

3. When ready to bake, preheat oven to 390 Fahrenheit or 200 Celsius.

4. Grease a loaf pan with addition oil of your choice before pouring the batter into the loaf pan.

5. Once the batter is in the loaf pan, shape the dough to resemble a smooth, curved top.

6. Bake the bread for 50 minutes or up until an hour. Remove the pan and remove the loaf right away.

Breakfast Ten - Eggs and Toast

Nutritional Information Per Serving (Eggs): 100 Calories, 8 grams of Fat, 3 grams of Carbs, 12 grams of Protein

Time: 7-8 minutes

Serving Size: 3 servings

Ingredients:

For the Eggs:

- 15 oz firm tofu, drained

- ½ teaspoon onion powder

- ½ teaspoon garlic powder

- ¼ teaspoon turmeric powder

- 1 tablespoon nutritional yeast

- 1 tablespoon almond milk

- Himalayan salt and black pepper to preference

For the Toast:

- Toast vegan store-bought bread or bake homemade bread using the instructions from *Breakfast Nine.*

Directions:

1. In a non-stick skillet add all egg ingredients and sauté over medium heat. Use a spatula to break up the tofu

into scramble-like pieces. This step should take about five to six minutes.

2. Serve the eggs with toast or any other additional vegan toppings.

Breakfast Eleven - Chickpea Skillet

Nutritional Information Per Serving: 425 Calories, 30 grams of Fat, 45 grams of Carbs, 19 grams of Protein

Time: 20 minutes

Serving Size: 2 servings

Ingredients:

- 2 medium potatoes, diced

- 2 tablespoons olive oil

- ½ teaspoon garlic powder

- 1 bell pepper, diced

- 1 small red onion, diced

- ½ cup chickpeas, drained and rinsed

- 1 handful fresh baby spinach

- 1 avocado, pitted and sliced

- 1 medium tomatoes, diced

- sea salt and black pepper to preference

Directions:

1. In a large pot, bring water to a boil. Add in potatoes and cook for 5 minutes. Drain potatoes.

2. In a cast iron skillet, heat olive oil over medium heat.

3. Add potatoes and spices to the skillet and spread the potatoes evenly. Do not stir for at least 5 minutes.

4. After five minutes, stir potatoes. Then spread them evenly across the pan again. Leave them for another five minutes or until crispy.

5. Add chopped bell pepper, chickpeas, and onion to the skillet. Cook until peppers are soft, then add in the spinach.

6. Stir the mixture and allow the spinach to soften for one minute. Then serve with toppings.

Breakfast Twelve - Chocolate Overnight Oats

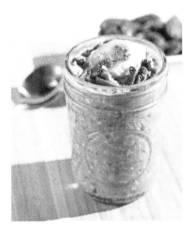

Nutritional Information Per Serving: 430 Calories, 27 grams of Fat, 45 grams of Carbs, 10 grams of Protein

Time: 5 minutes, (overnight recipe)

Serving Size: 1 serving

Ingredients:

- ½ cup rolled oats

- 1 tablespoon cocoa powder, unsweetened

- 1 tablespoon of chia seeds

- 1 tablespoon coconut oil, melted

- ½ cup coconut milk

- 1 tablespoon vegan chocolate chips

- vegan sweetener of choice

Directions:

1. In a glass mason jar, combine all ingredients before giving a vigorous shake.

2. Place in the refrigerator overnight and enjoy the next morning!

Breakfast Thirteen - Protein Smoothie Bowl

Nutritional Information Per Serving: 545 Calories, 33 grams of Fat, 58 grams of Carbs, 10 grams of Protein

Time: 5 minutes

Serving Size: 1 serving

Ingredients:

For the Smoothie:

- ½ avocado

- 1 tablespoon cocoa powder, unsweetened

- 1 teaspoon vanilla extract

- ½ cup coconut milk, unsweetened

- ½ cup ice

For the Toppings:

- ¼ cup almonds, sliced

- 1 tablespoon vegan chocolate chips

- ¼ cup blueberries

Directions:

1. Add all smoothie ingredients to a high-powered blender and blend until smooth. Create a thick, icy consistency.

2. Pour into a wide bowl.

2. Sprinkle toppings on top of the smoothie and eat with a spoon.

Lunch Recipes

Lunch One - Caesar Salad

Nutritional Information Per Serving: 500 Calories, 52 grams of Fat, 42 grams of Carbs, 13 grams of Protein

Time: 30 minutes

Serving Size: 4 servings

Ingredients:

- 2 cups sourdough bread, crumbled/cubed

- 2 tablespoons avocado oil

- 4 cups kale

- 2 cups arugula

- 2 avocados, pitted and diced

- ⅓ cup tahini

- 2 lemons, squeezed into juice

- 1 tablespoon apple cider vinegar

- 1 tablespoon olive oil

- 3 cloves garlic, diced

- sea salt and black pepper to preference

Directions:

1. Preheat oven to 350 Fahrenheit or 177 Celsius. Line a baking sheet with parchment paper.

2. Combine the bread, avocado oil, garlic powder, salt and pepper in a bowl. Mix well.

3. Pour the bread onto the baking sheet.

4. Bake for 10 minutes. Remove pan from oven and stir bread.

5. Return the bread to oven for additional 10 minutes.

6. While the bread is cooking mix the arugula, kale, and avocado in a bowl. Place in the refrigerator until the salad is ready to be consumed.

7. In a mason jar or blender, place tahini, lemon juice, apple cider vinegar, olive oil, garlic, salt and pepper. Shake or blend until dressing is smooth. Add water to reach desired consistency.

8. When the croutons are complete, add everything to the salad and serve!

Lunch Two - Buffalo Chickpeas

Nutritional Information Per Serving: 230 Calories, 6 grams of Fat, 34 grams of Carbs, 10 grams of Protein

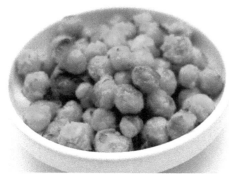

Time: 10 minutes

Serving Size: 2 servings

Ingredients:

- 1 can chickpeas, drained and rinsed

- 2 tablespoons tahini

- ¼ cup hot sauce

- 1 teaspoon onion powder

- 1 teaspoon smoked paprika

- 1 stalk celery, diced

Directions:

1. Place all ingredients except the celery in a food processor or blender and pulse to reach the desired consistency. You can also place all ingredients in a bowl and mash them together with a fork.

2. Stir in the chopped celery.

3. Serve on bread with fixings or over a salad. This can also be enjoyed plain or with crackers.

Lunch Three - Veg Wrap

Nutritional Information Per Serving: 550 Calories, 18 grams of Fat, 70 grams of Carbs, 18 grams of Protein

Time: 5 minutes

Serving Size: 1 serving

Ingredients:

- ½ cup cooked rice

- 1 whole wheat tortilla

- ½ avocado

- 2 tablespoons hummus (optional)

- ¼ cucumber, sliced

- ½ carrot stalk, sliced

- ½ cup black beans, drained and rinsed

Directions:

1. Prepare the rice and chop vegetables.

2. Place everything in tortilla along with your favorite vegan dressing. The Cesar dressing prepared for *Lunch One* is an excellent option.

Lunch Four- Egg Salad

Nutritional Information Per Serving: 255 Calories, 20 grams of Fat, 8 grams of Carbs, 14 grams of Protein

Time: 10 minutes

Serving Size: 4 servings

Ingredients:

- 1 block tofu, medium firm

- 6 tablespoons vegan mayonnaise

- 2 tablespoons nutritional yeast

- 2 teaspoons yellow mustard

- ¼ teaspoon turmeric

- 1 medium onion, chopped (optional)

- 4 stalks celery (chopped)

- Himalayan salt and black pepper to preference

Directions:

1. Drain and lightly press tofu to remove as much water as possible.

2. Combine all ingredients except onion and celery.

3. Use a spatula to mash everything together.

4. Fold in celery and onion.

5. Serve with bread, crackers, or over salad.

Lunch Five- Lunch Tacos

Nutritional Information Per Serving: 525 Calories, 21 grams of Fat, 70 grams of Carbs, 23 grams of Protein

Time: 5 minutes

Serving Size: 1 serving

Ingredients:

- ¼ cup black beans, drained and rinsed

- ½ avocado, pitted and diced

- ½ cup corn

- 2 tablespoons lime juice

- ⅓ cup cilantro, roughly chopped

- ¼ cup hummus

- 3 small corn tortillas

Directions:

1. Microwave or use a skillet to warm beans, corn, and tortillas.

2. Spread the hummus onto the tortillas evenly.

3. Add the remaining toppings and serve.

Lunch Six - Protein Bowl

Nutritional Information Per Serving: 600 Calories, 27 grams of Fat, 75 grams of Carbs, 19 grams of Protein

Time: 5 minutes

Serving Size: 1 serving

Ingredients:

- 4 cups raw spinach

- ½ cup chickpeas

- 1 cup quinoa, cooked

- ½ avocado

- ½ cup carrots, finely shredded

- 1 small red onion, diced

- 2 tablespoons olive oil

- 2 tablespoons apple cider vinegar

- sea salt and black pepper to preference

Directions:

1. Assemble the bowl by mixing everything together or strategically placing on the sides.

2. Drizzle the olive oil, apple cider vinegar, salt, and pepper over the top. You can also use your favorite vegan dressing if preferred and omit the oil.

Lunch Seven - Pesto Panini

Nutritional Information Per Serving: 400 Calories, 21 grams of Fat, 38 grams of Carbs, 14 grams of Protein

Time: 15 minutes

Serving Size: 1 serving

Ingredients:

For the Sandwich:
- ½ cup mushrooms, sliced

- 1 small onion, sliced

- ¼ cup red bell peppers, finely chopped

- 1 teaspoon of olive oil

- 2 pieces of sourdough bread

For the Sauce:
- ¼ cup fresh basil leaves

- ⅔ cup macadamia nuts, raw

- 1 teaspoon garlic powder

- 2 teaspoons nutritional yeast

- ½ tablespoon olive oil

- sea salt and black pepper to preference

Directions:

1. To prepare the sauce, place all ingredients into a food processor. Blend until smooth.

2. For the sandwich, place mushrooms, onion, red bell pepper, and small amount of oil into a skillet. Sauté until soft. This can be done the evening before and warmed up at work if necessary.

3. Toast or heat the bread.

4. Add vegetables and sauce to bread and serve as a sandwich.

Lunch Eight - Pasta Salad

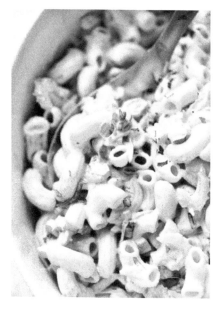

Nutritional Information Per Serving: 305 Calories, 6 grams of Fat, 45 grams of Carbs, 15 grams of Protein

Time: 20 minutes

Serving Size: 3 servings

Ingredients:

For the Salad:

- 5 oz dry pasta

- ½ red bell pepper, chopped

- 1 medium onion, chopped

- 2 small tomatoes, diced

- ¼ cucumber, diced

- ½ cup dill pickles, chopped

Dressing:

- 1½ cups white beans, drained and rinsed

- ¼ cup oat milk

- 2 tablespoons hulled hemp seeds

- 2 teaspoons of garlic powder

- ½ tablespoons lemon juice

- ½ tablespoon apple cider vinegar

Directions:

1. Cook pasta via the instructions on the packaging. Drain when finished.

2. In a blender or food processor add all dressing ingredients and blend until smooth.

3. Add the dressing, noodles, and chopped vegetables into a large bowl and mix well. Refrigerate until cold and serve.

Lunch Nine - Stuffed Sweet Potatoes

Nutritional Information Per Serving: 270 Calories, 12 grams of Fat, 36 grams of Carbs, 6 grams of Protein

Time: 45 minutes

Serving Size: 2 servings

Ingredients:

- 1 large sweet potato

- ½ tablespoon avocado oil

- ¼ cup green bell pepper, chopped

- ¼ cup corn

- ¼ cup quinoa

- ½ cup black beans, drained and rinsed

- ½ tablespoon chili powder

- ¼ teaspoon smoked paprika

- ½ avocado, mashed

- hot sauce (optional)

Directions:

1. Preheat oven to 400 Fahrenheit or 205 Celsius.

2. Place sweet potatoes on baking sheet and bake for 40 minutes. Prick the outside of the sweet potato first.

3. Place avocado oil in a non-stick frying pan and add the rest of the ingredients except the avocado.

4. Sauté vegetables for a few minutes.

5. When sweet potatoes are complete, remove from oven and top with vegetables and avocado. Serve immediately or warm when ready to consume.

Lunch Ten - Stir Fry

Nutritional Information Per Serving: 300 Calories, 21 grams of Fat, 20 grams of Carbs, 10 grams of Protein

Time: 25 minutes

Serving Size: 3 servings

Ingredients:

- 1 small onion, chopped

- 2 teaspoons of garlic powder

- 4 cups broccoli florets

- 1 tablespoon ginger, grated

- 1 cup roasted cashews

- 2-3 tablespoons soy sauce

- 1 tablespoon coconut oil

- 1½ cup quinoa (cooked)

Directions:

1. Follow the instructions on package to cook quinoa. Set quinoa aside when finished.

2. In a skillet sauté the onion and broccoli until soft using a little oil to prevent burning.

3. Add in garlic, ginger, cashews, and soy sauce. Stir.

4. Pour over quinoa and enjoy.

Lunch Eleven - Chicken Salad

Nutritional Information Per Serving: 209 Calories, 9 grams of Fat, 26 grams of Carbs, 9 grams of Protein

Time: 15 minutes

Serving Size: 4 servings

Ingredients:

- ½ cup almonds, halved/chopped
- 15 oz chickpeas, drained and rinsed
- 2 celery stalks, roughly chopped
- ½ cup red grapes, halved
- ¼ cup dried cranberries
- ½ cup vegan mayo (or oil)
- 1 tablespoon apple cider vinegar
- salt and pepper to preference

Directions:

1. In a food processor or blender add in almonds, chickpeas, celery, and spices. Pulse until the desired consistency is reached.

2. Add the mixture to a bowl and fold in grapes, cranberries, vegan mayo, and apple cider vinegar.

3. Serve cold over bread or over a salad.

Lunch Twelve - Mushroom Soup

Nutritional Information Per Serving: 195 Calories, 14 grams of Fat, 13 grams of Carbs, 9 grams of Protein

Time: 35 minutes

Serving Size: 4 servings

Ingredients:

- 1 tablespoon olive oil

- 1 medium onion, chopped

- 2 tablespoons garlic, minced

- 1 tablespoon oregano

- 1 tablespoon dried basil

- 24 oz mushrooms, sliced

- 3 tablespoons soy sauce

- 1 can full-fat coconut milk

- sea salt and pepper to preference

Directions:

1. Add olive oil to a large soup pot and warm over medium heat.

2. Add in onions and all spices. Sauté for four minutes.

3. Add mushrooms and all spices listed.

4. Let everything simmer with the lid on for 10 minutes and stir every so often.

5. Remove the lid and simmer for 10 minutes.

6. Add coconut milk and simmer for an additional 10 minutes.

7. Remove from heat and serve warm.

Dinner Recipes

Dinner One - Broccoli Cheese Dish

Nutritional Information Per Serving: 380 Calories, 9 grams of Fat, 65 grams of Carbs, 10 grams of Protein

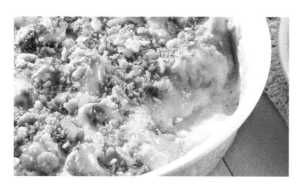

Time: 45 minutes

Serving Size: 6 servings

Ingredients:

- 2 cups brown rice, dry

- 1 teaspoon avocado oil

- 2 heads of broccoli, roughly chopped

- 1 medium onion, chopped

- 2 large tomatoes, peeled and cubed

- ½ cup carrots, chopped

- 2 cups water

- ⅔ cup cashews

- 1 tablespoon garlic, minced

- 2 tablespoons nutritional yeast

- sea salt and black pepper to preference

Directions:

1. In a large non-stick saucepan, cook rice using the directions on the packaging. When the rice is finished, set the rice into a large bowl to cool.

2. In the same pan used before, add olive oil and broccoli. Cook for two minutes over medium heat.

3. Add two tablespoons of water to the pan and steam broccoli for five minutes or until tender.

4. Remove broccoli when finished and set aside.

5. In the saucepan, add onion, potatoes, carrots, and 2 inches of water. Cover and bring water to a boil.

6. Reduce heat and simmer for 15 minutes or until vegetables are soft.

7. Add onions, potatoes and carrots to a blender.

8. Add 1 cup of water, cashews, spices, and nutritional yeast to the blender. Blend until smooth.

9. Add the broccoli and rice back to the saucepan. Cover with the sauce from the blender and stir.

10. Enjoy warm.

Dinner Two - Mushroom Stew

Nutritional Information Per Serving: 370 Calories, 13 grams of Fat, 48 grams of Carbs, 8 grams of Protein

Time: 1 hour 30 minutes (15 mins prep)

Serving Size: 2 servings

Ingredients:

For the Stew:

- 2 tablespoons olive oil

- 1 onion, chopped

- 1 tablespoon garlic, minced

- 2 cups vegetable broth

- 2 tablespoons flour

- 1 carrot, diced

- 1 large potato, cubed

- 2 cups mushrooms, stems removed

- ½ cup peas

- 1 tablespoon tomato paste

- 1 cup red wine

- Himalayan salt and black pepper to preference

Directions:

1. In a large pot, add 1 tablespoon olive oil, onions, and garlic. Simmer over medium heat for 10 minutes.

2. In a smaller pot, add 1 tablespoon of olive oil and flour over medium-low heat. Whisk until no lumps remain and slowly add in vegetable broth. Whisk until smooth.

3. Add carrots, potatoes, mushrooms, peas, tomato paste, salt, and pepper to the pot containing the onions/garlic. Stir.

4. Add red wine into the large pot containing the vegetables. Simmer on medium heat for three minutes.

5. Combine the small pot ingredients into the large stew pot. Stir.

6. Cover the pot and simmer on low heat for one hour.

7. Remove from heat, enjoy, and store any leftovers in the refrigerator.

Note: This recipe is best served over mashed potatoes, rice, or quinoa.

Dinner Three - Baked Ziti

Nutritional Information Per Serving: 376 Calories, 10 grams of Fat, 51 grams of Carbs, 15 grams of Protein

Time: 50 minutes

Serving Size: 4 servings

Ingredients:

For the Cheese:

- ¾ cups cashews, raw

- ¼ cup water

- 2 tablespoons lemon juice

- 2 tablespoons nutritional yeast

- 1 teaspoon garlic, minced

- ¼ teaspoon onion powder

- Himalayan salt and pepper to preference

The Ziti:

- ½ pound ziti noodles (vegan)

- 1 jar marinara sauce (12.5 ounces)

- ½ bag vegan shredded cheese

Directions:

1. Preheat oven to 375 degrees or 190 degrees Celsius. Grease a nine-by-thirteen casserole dish.

2. Soak the cashews in boiling hot water for five minutes. Drain and place in blender when finished.

3. Add water, lemon juice, nutritional yeast, garlic, onion powder, salt, and pepper to the blender.

4. Blend until smooth and creamy.

5. Prepare the pasta using the directions on the package.

6. When the noodles are finished, pour them into the casserole dish.

7. Pour marinara sauce over the noodles and stir.

8. Sprinkle vegan cheese over the top.

9. Place dish into oven and bake uncovered for 25 minutes.

Dinner Four - Vegan Chili

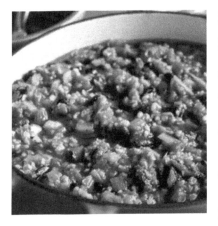

Nutritional Information Per Serving: 390 Calories, 8 grams of Fat, 55 grams of Carbs, 28 grams of Protein

Time: 40 minutes

Serving Size: 64 servings

Ingredients:

- 14 ounces taco meat (see recipe from *Lunch 21*)

- 1 medium onion, diced

- 2 tablespoon garlic, minced

- 2 28-oz cans crushed tomatoes

- 2 15-oz cans black beans, drained and rinsed

- 1 15-oz can kidney beans, drained and rinsed

- 1 cup water

- 3 tablespoons chili powder

- 1 teaspoon smoked paprika

- ¼ teaspoon cayenne pepper

- 1 tablespoon cocoa powder

- sea salt and pepper to preference

Directions:

1. Prepare taco meat using recipe from *Lunch 21*.

2. In a large pot, add a few tablespoons of water, onion, and garlic. Simmer over medium heat for five minutes.

3. Add all other chili ingredients excluding the taco meat. Stir.

4. Bring to a boil and then lower heat to low.

5. Simmer for 20 minutes and stir occasionally.

6. Stir in taco meat.

7. Serve with tortilla chips, hot sauce, chives, tomatoes, avocado or any other desired toppings.

Dinner Five - Alfredo Sauce Recipe

Nutritional Information Per Serving: 435 Calories, 19 grams of Fat, 50 grams of Carbs, 16 grams of Protein

Time: 15 minutes

Serving Size: 3 servings

Ingredients:

- ¾ cups cashews, raw

- 1 tablespoon olive oil

- ½ medium sized onion

- 1 teaspoon garlic, minced

- 1 cup cashew milk

- 4 tablespoons nutritional yeast

- ½ tablespoon lemon juice

- Himalayan salt and pepper to preference

Directions:

1. Boil 2 cups of water and pour over cashews in a glass bowl. Allow them to soak for five minutes.

2. In a skillet, add oil, onion, and garlic. Sauté for five minutes.

3. Drain the cashews and place in a high-speed blender.

4. Add the onions, garlic, cashew milk, nutritional yeast, lemon juice, salt, and pepper. Blend until smooth.

5. Return sauce to the pan to warm, or store until you're ready to consume.

Note: This recipe makes a great addition to pastas, potatoes, and other dishes.

Dinner Six - Fajitas

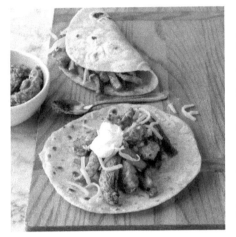

Nutritional Information Per Serving: 120 Calories, 5 grams of Fat, 12 grams of Carbs, 3 grams of Protein

Time: 35 minutes

Serving Size: 3 servings

Ingredients:

- 2 cups cauliflower, in florets

- 1 red pepper, sliced

- 1 green pepper, sliced

- 1 small onion, sliced

- 3 tablespoons olive oil

- ½ tablespoon chili powder

- ½ teaspoon cumin

- ½ teaspoon onion powder

- sea salt and pepper to preference

Directions:

1. Preheat oven to 425 Fahrenheit or 218 Celsius. Line a sheet pan with parchment paper.

2. In a large bowl, mix all spices together.

3. Toss in all vegetables and olive oil. Mix well to evenly coat the vegetables.

4. Add the mixture to a sheet pan and roast for 25 minutes or until vegetables have crispy edges.

5. Serve with tortillas or over a salad. Serve with toppings like guacamole, hot sauce, and rice if preferred.

Dinner Seven - Meatless Meatloaf

Nutritional Information Per Serving: 305 Calories, 17 grams of Fat, 28 grams of Carbs, 10 grams of Protein

Time: 1 hour

Serving Size: 4 servings

Ingredients:

- ½ tablespoon olive oil

- 1 small onion, roughly chopped

- 4 ounces of mushrooms, finely chopped

- 1 small carrot, peeled and diced

- ¾ cup walnuts

- 1 cup cooked lentils

- 1 tablespoon ground flaxseed

- 1 tablespoon ketchup

- 1 tablespoon Worcestershire sauce

- ¼ cup breadcrumbs

- sea salt and pepper to preference

Directions:

1. Preheat oven to 350 Fahrenheit or 177 Celsius. Line a standard loaf pan with parchment paper.

2. Add olive oil, onions, mushrooms, and carrots to a large pan.

3. Sauté on medium heat for five minutes. After, set aside.

4. Add walnuts to a food processor and pulse a few times. Add in lentils and pulse a few more times.

5. In a large bowl, add the lentils, walnuts, vegetables, flaxseed, ketchup, Worcestershire sauce, salt, and pepper. Mix well.

6. Fold in breadcrumbs.

7. Transfer mixture to loaf pan and press the mixture to even. Cover with foil.

8. Bake for 30 minutes.

9. Remove from oven and serve warm. Add additional ketchup if desired.

Dinner Eight - Veggie Burger

Nutritional Information Per Burger: 220 Calories, 6 grams of Fat, 30 grams of Carbs, 9 grams of Protein

Time: 45 minutes

Serving Size: 12 burgers

Ingredients:

- ¼ cup ground flax

- ½ cup water

- 3 cups black beans, drained and rinsed

- 1 cup cashews

- 1½ cup rice

- ½ cup parsley

- 1½ cup shredded carrots

- ⅓ cup green onions, chopped

- 1 cup breadcrumbs

- 2 tablespoons chili powder

- 1 tablespoon garlic, minced

- 1 teaspoon sea salt

Directions:

1. Preheat oven to 350 Fahrenheit or 177 Celsius. Line two baking sheets with parchment paper.

2. In a cup, add flaxseed and water. Put in refrigerator.

3. In a large bowl add black beans and use a fork to mash them.

4. Place cashews in a food processor and pulse a few times. Add them to the large bowl.

5. Remove flax water from refrigerator and add to the large bowl. Mix well.

6. Form patties. You should have about 12.

7. Place on parchment paper.

8. Bake for 20 minutes. Then flip the patties and bake for an additional 15 minutes.

9. Allow cooling before removing patties.

10. Enjoy on a bun, over a salad, and with your favorite toppings.

Dinner Nine - Tuna Salad

Nutritional Information Per Serving: 280 Calories, 7 grams of Fat, 41 grams of Carbs, 13 grams of Protein

Time: 10 minutes

Serving Size: 3 servings

Ingredients:

- 1 15-oz can chickpeas, drained and rinsed

- 1 medium dill pickle, chopped

- 1 celery stalk, roughly chopped

- 2 tablespoons vegan mayo

- ½ tablespoon soy sauce

Directions:

1. In a bowl, use a fork to mash chickpeas. You can have a smooth texture or leave some beans whole.

2. Add in remaining ingredients and stir.

3. Place mixture in the refrigerator until ready to be consumed.

Note: This recipe should be served over a bed of lettuce, with crackers, or as a sandwich.

Dinner Ten - Instant Pot Pasta

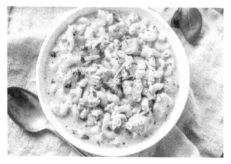

Nutritional Information Per Serving: 325 Calories, 4 grams of Fat, 60 grams of Carbs, 18 grams of Protein

Time: 20 minutes

Serving Size: 5 servings

Ingredients:

- 1 tablespoon olive oil

- 1 small onion, diced

- 1 tablespoon garlic, minced

- 2 cups lentils, cooked

- 2 cups water

- 8 oz spaghetti

- 1 jar marinara sauce (25.5) ounces

Directions:

1. Press the sauté button on instant pot.

2. When hot add olive oil, onion, and garlic. Cook for 4 minutes. Stir occasionally.

3. Add salt, pepper, and cooked lentils. Stir.

4. Turn off the sauté.

5. Pour in water and use a spatula to make sure nothing is sticking to the bottom.

6. Break the noodles in half, and add to instant pot.

7. Pour marinara sauce over everything and close the cover. Don't stir.

8. Set instant pot to high pressure and cook for 9 minutes.

9. Do a quick release and then stir everything together. Enjoy!

Dinner Eleven - Peanut Tofu with Rice

Nutritional Information Per Serving: 460 Calories, 20 grams of Fat, 42 grams of Carbs, 19 grams of Protein

Time: 30 minutes

Serving Size: 3 servings

Ingredients:

Tofu:

- 1 block of tofu, extra-firm (vacuum sealed if possible)

- 1 tablespoon soy sauce

- 1 tablespoon cornstarch

Rice:

- ½ cup rice, dry

- ¼ cup canned coconut milk

- ¾ cup water

- sea salt to preference

Sauce:

- ¼ cup peanut butter

- ½ cup canned coconut milk

- 1 tablespoon soy sauce

- 1 teaspoon ginger, grater

- 1 teaspoon garlic, minced

- 1 tablespoon lime juice

Directions:

1. Press tofu and remove as much water as possible if the pack is not vacuum sealed.

2. Preheat oven to 400 Fahrenheit or 204 Celsius. Line a baking sheet with parchment paper and spray with oil.

3. Slice tofu into medium-sized cubes. Place them into a large bowl.

4. Add soy sauce and stir gently, followed by the cornstarch.

5. Place tofu cubes onto baking sheet and cook for 25 minutes. The tofu should appear crispy and golden brown.

6. In a pot, add rice, coconut milk, water, and salt. Bring water to a boil.

7. Turn to low heat and simmer the rice for 18 minutes.

8. In a large pan, add all the sauce ingredients and simmer over medium heat. Stir frequently. Allow the sauce to simmer for 10 minutes.

9. Add the tofu to the sauce and serve over rice!

Dinner Twelve - Spicy Tahini Pasta

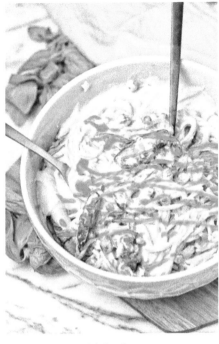

Nutritional Information Per Serving: 325 Calories, 7 grams of Fat, 56 grams of Carbs, 15 grams of Protein

Time: 25 minutes

Serving Size: 4 servings

Ingredients:

For the Sauce:

- ¼ cup tahini

- ½ water

- ½ habanero pepper, seeded

- 1 tablespoon garlic, minced

- ½ lemon, juiced

- sea salt and pepper to preference

For the Pasta

- 8 ounces linguini pasta, cooked

- 2 cups green peas, steamed

- 4 cups mushrooms, sliced and sautéed

- a dab of oil for frying

Directions:

1. Prepare noodles and peas according to their packages and set aside.

2. In a pan, sauté mushrooms over medium heat for five minutes or until soft. Use a dab of oil if necessary.

3. In a separate pan, add garlic and habanero peppers. Sauté for 3 minutes.

4. Add all the sauce ingredients, including garlic and peppers, to a blender. Blend until smooth.

5. Add the sauce to the pan containing mushrooms. Stir.

6. Add in pasta and stir to combine all ingredients.

7. Enjoy and serve warm!

Snacks

Snack 1 - Spinach and Artichoke Dip

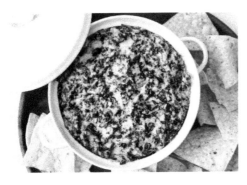

Nutritional Information Per Serving: 75 Calories, 6 grams of Fat, 5 grams of Carbs, 3 grams of Protein

Time: 20 minutes

Serving Size: 10 servings

Ingredients:

- 1 tablespoon avocado oil

- 3 cloves garlic, diced

- 12 oz marinated artichoke hearts

- 4 cups baby spinach, chopped

- ¼ cup vegan mayo

- 8 oz vegan cream cheese

- ½ teaspoon onion powder

- sea salt and black pepper to preference

Directions:

1. Preheat oven to 400 Fahrenheit or 205 Celsius.

2. Heat the avocado oil in a pan over medium heat. Add garlic, artichoke hearts, and spinach. Simmer for three minutes.

3. Add cream cheese, mayo, onion powder, salt, and pepper. Mix well.

4. Add the mixture to a baking dish and place under the broiler for five minutes.

5. Remove and enjoy warm.

Note: This recipe is best served with crackers or tortilla chips. This recipe is excellent to bring to parties.

Snack Two - Buffalo Dip

Nutritional Information Per Serving: 190 Calories, 16 grams of Fat, 10 grams of Carbs, 6 grams of Protein

Time: 40 minutes

Serving Size: 10 servings

Ingredients:

- 2 cups raw cashews

- 1 cup water

- 3 tablespoons lemon juice

- 2 teaspoons onion powder

- 1 teaspoon garlic powder

- 1 cup buffalo/hot sauce

- 14 oz artichoke hearts, drained

- sea salt and black pepper to preference

Directions:

1. Preheat oven to 375 Fahrenheit or 190 degrees Celsius.

2. Pour boiling hot water over cashews and allow them to soak for 5 minutes. Drain and place in blender when finished.

3. Add water, lemon juice, garlic powder, onion powder, salt and pepper to the blender containing the cashews. Blend until smooth.

4. Add buffalo sauce and artichoke hearts to the blender. Pulse until the artichoke hearts are broken down. You'll want to leave some texture to the dip.

5. Transfer to baking dish and bake for 30 minutes.

Note: This recipe is best served with celery sticks, carrot sticks, tortilla chips, crackers, or bread.

Snack Three - Potato Wedges

Nutritional Information Per Serving: 250 Calories, 6 grams of Fat, grams of Carbs, 10 grams of Protein

Time: 45 minutes

Serving Size: 6 servings

Ingredients:

- 4 medium potatoes

- 2 tablespoons avocado oil

- 2 teaspoons of garlic powder

- 2 teaspoons onion powder

- 1 teaspoon smoked paprika

- Himalayan salt and pepper to preference

Directions:

1. Preheat oven to 425 Fahrenheit or 218 Celsius. Grease a large baking pan with a dab of oil.

2. Clean potatoes and remove dirt.

3. Slice potatoes in half and then into wedges.

4. In a large Ziplock bag, place potatoes and all other ingredients. Shake the bag to evenly coat the potatoes.

5. Spread potatoes oven baking pan and bake for 35 minutes. Flip and stir the wedges halfway through.

6. Remove wedges when golden brown and tender. Serve warm with your favorite vegan sauce.

Desserts Recipes

Dessert One - Blondies

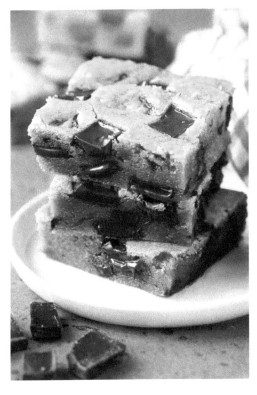

Nutritional Information Per Serving: 300 Calories, 13 grams of Fat, 42 grams of Carbs, 8 grams of Protein

Time: 40 minutes

Serving Size: 9 servings

Ingredients:

- 1 15-oz can chickpeas, rinsed and drained

- ¾ cup brown sugar

- ⅓ cup creamy peanut butter

- 1 teaspoon vanilla extract

- ¼ cup almond flour

- ¼ teaspoon baking soda

- ½ teaspoon baking powder

- ¾ cup vegan chocolate chips

- pinch of Himalayan salt

Directions:

1. Preheat oven to 350 Fahrenheit or 177 Celsius. Line an 8 x 8 pan with parchment paper.

2. Add all ingredients to a food processor except for the chocolate chips. Blend until smooth.

3. Fold in half of the chocolate chips.

4. Pour batter into the pan. Sprinkle the rest of the chocolate chips on top.

5. Bake for 27 minutes.

6. Let the blondies cool before serving.

Dessert Two - Peanut Butter Cups

Nutritional Information Per Serving: 215 Calories, 16 grams of Fat, 22 grams of Carbs, 5 grams of Protein

Time: 30 minutes

Serving Size: 12 servings

Ingredients:

- 2 cups vegan chocolate chips

- ½ cup peanut butter

- 4 tablespoons powdered sugar

- pinch of salt

Directions:

1. Line muffin tray with paper liners. You will need 12 liners.

2. Microwave 1 cup of chocolate chips in a microwave-safe bowl for one minute.

3. Stir and repeat in five second increments to prevent burning. Stir frequently.

4. Scoop ½ tablespoon of the chocolate and place into each liner. Use a spoon to create an even surface and bring the chocolate up onto the sides of the liner.

5. Repeat step 4 until each liner is filled.

6. Freeze the muffin pan for 10 minutes.

7. In a bowl, add peanut butter, salt, and powdered sugar. Mix well until a dough is formed.

8. Remove pan from freezer and place a tablespoon of peanut butter into each cup. Press down on the dough with a spoon to create a smooth surface.

9. Freeze pan for additional 10 minutes.

10. Melt remaining chocolate chips. Spoon chocolate evenly over the now frozen peanut butter mixture.

11. Remove the liners and store in the refrigerator to prevent melting until ready to be consumed.

Dessert Three - Chocolate Mug Cake

Nutritional Information Per Serving: 320 Calories, 16 grams of Fat, 42 grams of Carbs, 5 grams of Protein

Time: 1 minute

Serving Size: 1 serving

Ingredients:

- 2 tablespoons all-purpose flour
- 2 tablespoons cocoa powder
- 2 tablespoons sugar
- ¼ teaspoon baking powder
- 1 tablespoon coconut oil
- 3 tablespoons coconut milk
- ½ teaspoon pure vanilla extract
- 2 tablespoons vegan chocolate chips
- pinch of Himalayan salt

Directions:

1. In a microwave safe mug, add flour, cocoa powder, sugar, salt, and baking powder. Stir well.

2. Pour in the oil, milk, and vanilla into the mug. Mix well then add chocolate chips on top.

3. Microwave for 40 seconds and serve immediately.

Dessert Four - Ice Cream

Nutritional Information Per Serving (2 Scoops): 140 Calories, 15 grams of Fat, 4 grams of Carbs, 3 grams of Protein

Time: 5 minutes

Serving Size: 10 servings

Ingredients:

- 2 14-oz cans full-fat coconut milk

- ½ cup soaked cashews, raw

- ⅓ cup cocoa powder

- 1 teaspoon vanilla extract

- pinch of sea salt

- sweetener of choice

Directions:

1. In a blender, place all ingredients and blend until smooth.

2. Place the mixture in a plastic Ziploc bag and freeze until solid.

3. When ready to consume, allow the ice cream to thaw slightly before serving.

Preworkout Recipes

Preworkout: One - Peanut Butter Toast

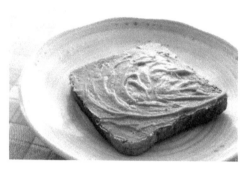

Nutritional Information Per Serving: 255 Calories, 13 grams of Fat, 26 grams of Carbs, 9 grams of Protein

Time: 5 minutes

Serving Size: 1 serving

Ingredients:

- 1 tablespoon peanut butter

- 1 piece of hearty toast

- ½ banana

- 1 teaspoon chia seeds

Directions:

1. Assemble the toast by toasting the bread, adding the peanut butter, slicing the banana on top, and sprinkling over chia seeds.

Preworkout: Two - Tropical Smoothie

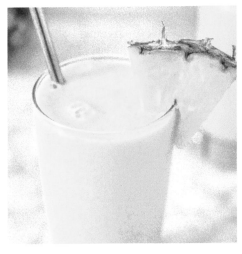

Nutritional Information Per Serving: 455 Calories, 17 grams of Fat, 60 grams of Carbs, 17 grams of Protein

Time: 5 minutes

Serving Size: 1 serving

Ingredients:

- 1 cup frozen mango

- ½ cup pineapple

- 3 cups kale

- 2 tablespoons hemp seeds

- ¼ cup orange juice

- 1 cup coconut milk

- pinch of Himalayan salt

Directions:

1. Add all ingredients into a high-speed blender and blend
   until smooth.

Preworkout: Three - Apple Slices and Almond Butter

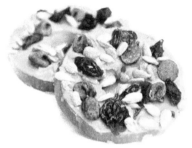

Nutritional Information Per Serving: 162 Calories, 18 grams of Fat, 25 grams of Carbs, 8 grams of Protein

Time: 5 minutes

Serving Size: 1 serving

Ingredients:

- 1 medium apple

- 2 tablespoons almond butter

Directions:

1. Wash and slice the apple before serving alongside almond butter.

Postworkout Recipes

Postworkout: One - BodyBuilding Smoothie

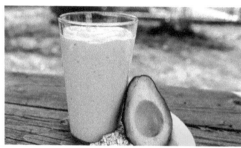

Nutritional Information Per Serving: 950 Calories, 28 grams of Fat, 154 grams of Carbs, 38 grams of Protein

Time: 5 minutes

Serving Size: 1 serving

Ingredients:

- 2 bananas

- 3 tablespoons chia seeds

- ½ cup chickpeas

- 2 tablespoons dried dates

- 1 tablespoon peanut butter

- 2 cups spinach

- dash of turmeric

- dash of black pepper

- 1 cup soymilk

Directions:

1. Add all ingredients to a high-speed blender and blend until smooth.

Postworkout: Two - Spinach Salad with Tempeh

Nutritional Information Per Serving: 460 Calories, 29 grams of Fat, 29 grams of Carbs, 20 grams of Protein

Time: 15 minutes

Serving Size: 1 serving

Ingredients:

- 3 cups spinach

- 3 oz tempeh, cooked

- ½ cup blueberries

- ¼ cup pecans

Directions:

1. Assemble the salad and add your favorite dressing.

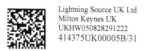